Table of Contents

Lifestyle Changes To Make Your Dream Come True

The start of the year marks a new beginning, characterized with new resolutions, bigger plans, and strategies to accomplish a set goals. According to findings on Statista, most people resolve to eat healthier, exercise more, and lose weight. One of the items on your to do list may be to learn how to lose 50 lb in 2 months, so here is everything you need to know to make your dream come true.

Wondering how to lose 50 lb in 2 months? There are hundreds, if not thousands of resources that you may come across, all approaching this issue from unique angles. If you are new to weight loss, these resources may overwhelm you due to the diversity of the ideas brought forth. Despite this, the steps to be followed in pursuit of a 50 lb weight loss in 2 months can be summed up into one fact. Expert recommended weight loss calls for a suitable, healthy, manageable, and realistic plan that you can follow to the end.

How To Lose 50 lb In 2 Months

How long does it take to lose 50 pounds? 50 lbs is equal to about 22.7 kilograms. The purpose of this article is to equip you with information on how to lose 50 pounds in 2 months. According to the Centre for Disease Control and Prevention, among other credible sources, one could lose about 1-2 pounds a week, which means that the recommended time frame to lose 50 lbs is between 25-50 weeks (7 months to 1 year). Keep in mind that everyone is different and so among people following the same weight loss routine there will be different rates of fat lost, depending on their genetics, gender, and age, among other factors.

Learning how to lose 50 pounds in 2 months may sound impossible, but some people have tried it and succeeded. Whether you are preparing for an event or you just want to look good, you can lose 50 pounds in 2 months, depending on the effort you put into the process and your commitment to the weight loss program. Remember, weight loss is a journey in which every step counts, therefore, focus should not be on how much, by what time, but in making lifestyle changes that will help you shed those unwanted pounds reasonably and maintain a healthy weight.

You also need to be aware of the other contributing factors to the amount of weight you can drop in a short period. For instance, the heavier you are, the easier it is to lose 50 pounds in 2 months because of a greater mass than others, therefore biophysics favours you when you exercise.

Lifestyle Changes To Help You Lose Weight

The basic weight loss equation is that calorie intake should be less than calories burnt. This means that to get to your ideal weight, you should decrease the number of calories you eat and increase calories burnt. Calorie intake is determined by your diet, and calories burnt mostly depends on your level of physical activity.

Diet Tweaks That Can Help You Shed Weight In Two Months

You are what you eat, therefore, replacing lousy eating habits with a healthy diet is the first step in learning how to lose weight in a month or more. According to Britannica, the average human body comprises less than 1% carbohydrates, 6% minerals, 16% protein, 16% fat, and a more significant water percentage (about 62%). Although these percentages vary depending on the individual, it should paint a clear picture of the macronutrients you need to invest in for a healthy body.

There are many traditional and modern diets such as the Caveman, Military, Subway, and Cabbage Soup diet. Despite their differences in origin and ingredients, these meal plans may help you lose weight as long as you identify the right one. Better still, your dietician may create an eating plan that is tailored for you. Remember, what you eat and how much you eat matters. Here are some eating tips that will help you lose weight:

1. Incorporate More Fruits And Vegetables In Your Meals

Fruits and vegetables have long been associated with several health benefits and nutritional value. They have plenty of water, low calories, and higher fiber content, in addition to numerous vitamins and minerals.They also contain a rich base of antioxidants, which help boost the body's immune system.

According to research, increasing your fruit and vegetable consumption may help with weight loss and body weight maintenance. Some of the fruits and vegetables that help lose weight and burn stubborn belly fat include:

• Grapefruit

• Kiwi

• Guava

• Tomatoes

• Apples

• Pumpkin

• Cauliflower

• Cucumber

• Kale

• Broccoli

• Asparagus

Fruits and vegetables can fit many recipes for your weight loss diet plan. For instance, you can blend carrots with an apple to create a fresh, healthy, nutritious drink. You can also grill spinach with skinless chicken breast for a healthy lunch.

2. Avoid Overeating

Eating more than is necessary is a big step backward when trying to lose 50 pounds in 2 months because it is one of the main reasons people gain weight quickly. There are 2 types of overeating-eating when there is no physiological need, and eating too much when hungry. Before you go down that route, you can adopt a few strategies to help you prevent or slow down the chances of overeating.

- Break free from screens, phones, or laptops while eating, and take a moment to enjoy your meals. We eat with our eyes too, so paying attention to what you put in your mouth will help you know when you are satisfied and stop, unlike when your attention is divided.

• Watch out for sugar, salt, and other seasonings that make your big plate of food delicious. If you want a sweet snack in between the meals, take a small bite at a time. Eat snacks that are unsalted or low in sodium.

• Avoid eating unless you are truly hungry. People may eat just because they are bored, craving, emotional for example angry or stressed. It would help if you consulted a psychologist to help you manage your inner self instead of eating to suppress your emotions.

3. Track Your Calories

Losing 50 lb in two months means losing about 6.25 lb per week, meaning you will have to burn over 2500 calories on top of what you consume every day. Counting your calorie intake may be tedious and tiresome, but it is key when it comes to losing 5 pounds in a week. A simple solution is to create a weekly meal plan listing all the meals you will have that week and how many calories each contains. Doing so helps plan out your entire week and gives you more details on what the diet contains or what might be missing.

The second approach is to use online resources to calculate how many calories your body needs to lose or maintain. Many online calculators, apps, and websites automatically process such data to help you understand your current situation. All you need to do is feed the calorie calculator with variables such as height, weight, and activity level, and the calculator will do the rest.

On average, you also need to consume 300 calories in every meal (3 main meals and 2 snacks) so that you will have consumed approximately 1,500 at the end of the day, which is lower than the daily required calorie intake for men (2,500 kcal) and women (2,000 kcal). Having less calories means the body will tap into its reserves to get energy, and this will lead to weight loss.

4. Drink Lots Of Water

Water plays a pivotal role in the body. It keeps your systems in perfect health by maintaining your body's electrolyte balance, protecting organs and tissues, keeps you hydrated, and aids in digestion, among other roles.

You need to drink slightly more than two liters of water a day on a weight loss diet a day, preferably two glasses 20 minutes before each meal. Research reveals that people who drink plenty of water on a hypocaloric diet (caloric deficit), show a 44% decrease in weight when compared to those who do not. Plain water contains zero calories, but if you do not like its tastelessness, you can squeeze a fresh lemon, lime, or try a few slices of cucumber to make it tastier.

5. Intermittent Fasting

Intermittent fasting is one of the most common methods of weight loss. It involves partially eating or completely refraining from eating for a specific period. It is a cycle revolving around eating and fasting periods, typically within an 8-10 hour window. According to Sue Ryskamp, a Michigan Medicine dietitian, your insulin levels go down during the fasting period, helping the body burn fat. During this period, your body releases its glucose stores as energy, which leads to weight loss.

There are several variations of the intermittent diet to choose from. However, determining the best approach depends on you- it is advisable to choose a diet plan and time frame that works for you.

The 5:2 diet

5:2 diet involves eating for five days and then fast for two non-consecutive days. For the 5 eating days, you do not have to worry about calorie restriction. But during the fasting period, men can target approximately 600 calories while women can aim for 500 calories. You can also choose which days to eat and which ones to fast since there is no pattern to adhere to. The diet focuses more on when you eat than what you eat.

The Warrior Diet

The Warrior diet is considered an extreme form of intermittent fasting whereby a person survives on a few fruit and vegetable servings within 20 hours and later eats a mega meal at night. When eating a large meal at night, always remember to include plenty of vegetables, proteins, and healthy fats such as avocado for replenishment. The Warrior diet is more friendly to people who are used to other intermittent fasting diets.

Alternate Day Fasting

Here, you get to choose whether to avoid food entirely on the fasting days or reduce caloric intake under the alternate-day fasting, say 500 calories. On the feeding day, one can choose how much to eat. Although alternate day fasting sounds excellent, you need to understand that it might seem a little bit extreme for beginners, and you might not be able to keep up. Also, you need to consult your doctor if you have any underlying medical conditions.

Other IF diets include 16:8 diet, 12-hour fast, Eat-Stop-Eat diet, and Meal skipping. Before proceeding with intermittent fasting, you need to be ready for some adverse side effects such as hunger, nausea, and insomnia. You may also face a hard time fitting in because intermittent fasting requires a lot of self-control to avoid the temptations of eating when fasting. But if you stay strong and stick to the diet, you could enjoy other benefits, such as a short-term intervention to type 2 diabetes and reduction of blood pressure among other risk factors for cardiovascular disease.

6. Avoid Drinking Too Much Alcohol And High-calorie Beverages

The human body is wired in such a way that it opts for the quickest energy source, and as long as there are more readily available energy sources other than fat, your body will obtain energy from them. Sodas, beer, energy drinks, and alcohol provide a faster and more accessible energy fuel than fat.

Drinking too much alcohol could frustrate your efforts to lose 50 pounds in 3 months or less. Alcohol is packed with carbs and calories from its composite additives and mixtures. Besides, alcohol is an appetite stimulant (leads to greater hunger and less satiety) that hinders your body from burning fat and encourages you to make bad meal choices. Science backs this with research that links heavy drinking with an astonishing transition from average weight to overweight . Therefore, staying away from alcohol could help prevent weight gain and prevent other health-related conditions such as liver disease, high blood pressure, and insulin resistance.

Note that drinking while trying to lose 50lb in 2 months is not bad unless it is overdone. If you must drink, take time to read through the composition of what you are consuming. According to nutritionist Amy Gorin, you should also watch out for what you mix your drink with because if you mix vodka with a high-calorie beverage, it could delay your progress.

Low-Calorie Alcohol Choices

Some low-calorie alcohol choices include:

- Champagne (90 calories)

- Vodka soda (96 calories)

- Rum and coke (97 calories)

- Whisky (105 calories)

- Gin & Tonic (115 calories)

- Pinot noir (Red Wine 123 calories)

Whether you intend to lose 50 pounds in 3 months, less or more, the best diet to adopt for is the one that works well for all your body parts, not just your arms, legs, or belly. A good diet provides all nutrients, and you can live with it for a long time without needing expensive supplements.

B. Physical Activities And Exercise For 50 Lb Weight Loss

Other than eating, physical activity is the other secret ingredient for a successful weight loss plan. Without it, your efforts in dietary changes may only lead you halfway there.

Cardio

Cardio, AKA aerobic exercises, are physical activities that increase your heart rate. They make your body consume oxygen and, in the process, help you burn more fat and calories. When it comes to weight loss, you can try several types of cardio exercises, including simple exercises such as swimming, walking, and cycling. Cardio exercises do not have to be actual workout routines because simpler activities like mopping can equally qualify as cardio.

If you are more into the actual cardio workout routines, you can try out the physically demanding exercises. But first, you need to determine which exercises you need to do to get the body type you are aiming for. For example, if you want a runner's body, go for the distant running cardio.

• Stationary bike workouts- A 185-pound person can burn 311 calories in 30 minutes at a moderate pace.

• Elliptical- Above moderate pace, a 180-pound man can burn 500-600 calories per hour.

- Rope jumping can help burn 500 calories in just 30 minutes.

- Rowing – A 180-pound guy can lose 800 calories per hour.

Strength Training

Strength training is a form of exercise where your muscles are worked against an opposing force—for example, lifting weights to increase your strength. Michaela Devries, an exercise physiologist at McMaster University, insists that strength training does a better job building muscle than cardio alone . Having more muscle means that your Basal Metabolic Rate (BMR) improves, and this means that your body will burn more calories at rest. Noam Tamir, the founder of TS Fitness, adds that the body breaks down muscle and recreates it in a process that requires energy. The more your muscles, the more the energy needed for these processes, increasing your metabolism. Some basic strength training exercises you could try out include:

- **Weight lifting**

- Push-ups, pull-ups, crunches, and leg squats

- Resistance bands

- Deadlifts

For better results, try combining strength training with cardio-strength training for 45-60 minutes three to four times a week helps prepare the body for aerobic exercise. Apart from diet and working out, remember to get enough sleep and manage your stress.

Healthy Weight Loss Per Week

As mentioned earlier, CDC recommends a healthy weight loss of 1-2 pounds a week for the best results. People who lose weight at this rate are more successful than others at keeping it off. Losing 50 lb in two months is almost three times the recommended weight loss per week. According to Mayo Clinic, losing too much weight too fast usually demands big changes in diet and workout plans, which could be unhealthy for your body. Even worse, it could lead to loss of water weight or lean muscle. Once you attain your target weight, it is essential to keep up with the exercises and maintain a healthy diet.

How long does it take to lose 30 pounds? The answer depends on the approach you intend to take and the time you're willing to sacrifice. For instance, if you decide to lose weight at the recommended rate (1-2 pounds a week), it could take between 4-8 months and 25 weeks to lose 50 pounds.

Final Thought

How to lose 50 lb in 2 months depends on your diet, level of physical activity, and other lifestyle changes. However, remember that although it may sound awesome to lose a tremendous amount of weight in a short span, there are adverse health impacts you should be aware of. Follow a healthy weight loss diet and workout routine that is sustainable. Get a green light from your doctor, nutritionist and personal trainer before engaging in any weight loss routine.

Diets are great, but your body will thank you if you supplement your healthy nutrition plan with a good workout.

Morning Drink For Weight Loss: 10 Morning Drinks To Cut Belly

Losing weight isn't a walk in the park. It is quite challenging and sometimes can be a nightmare. The process of shedding away pounds is gradual and obliges a combination of workouts with the right diet. While diet seems to imply what is on your plate, what is in your glass counts as well. So now, what is the best morning drink for weight loss?

When combined with healthy lifestyle changes, a morning detox drink for weight loss can promote the rate at which you shed pounds. It can also influence your health and energy levels for the day. Here is what you need to know about the best thing to drink in the morning for weight loss.

What To Drink In The Morning For Weight Loss?

According to Medical News Today, drinking the right beverage in the morning can go a long way in helping you control your appetite.

With a reduced appetite, you will consume fewer than usual calories for the day. If you are looking to add a fantastic beverage to your routine, here is what to drink first thing in the morning for weight loss.

1. Vegetable Juice

A vegetable drink is the best juice to drink in the morning for weight loss.

As you might know, fruit juices have been linked with weight gain. Drinking vegetable juice will give you the opposite effect.

In one study, subjects who drank about 16 ounces of low-sodium veggie juice while on a low-calorie diet lost a lot of weight compared with those who didn't.

According to the findings, the vegetable juice group shed more pounds due to their vegetable consumption and reduced carb intake. These two factors are essential when it comes to weight loss.

For the best results, consume whole vegetables rather than juiced ones, since they have high amounts of fibers that are often lost during the juicing process.

Most importantly, a vegetable juice contains fewer calories and will increase your daily vegetable intake. This will lead to weight loss.

2. Ginger Tea

Ginger is a spice used to add flavor to a lot of dishes. It is also used as herbal medicine to treat conditions such as colds, arthritis, and nausea.

Human and animal research has shown this flavourful root to be beneficial when it comes to weight loss.

One study found out that rats fed with high-fat meals supplemented with ginger powder for around four weeks had noticeable body weight reductions. The rats also had a significant improvement in HDL cholesterol levels, compared to those that did not consume ginger.

Another study in humans found that taking 2 grams of ginger powder dissolved in hot water as breakfast could increase the feeling of fullness. This resulted in decreased hunger and consumption of fewer calories per day.

The study also showed that ginger tea could increase the thermic effects of food (number of calories burned during digestion and absorption of food substances) by around 43 calories.

Although 43 calories isn't huge, taking ginger tea can enhance your weight loss through its satiating properties.

3. Green Tea

Green tea is the best tea to drink in the morning for weight loss. For a good reason, this tea is associated with health by many scientists.

The drink is packed with antioxidants and other powerful nutrients that promote weight loss.

Taking green tea in the morning has been shown by various studies to decrease body fat and overall weight.

A review of 14 pieces of research found out that people who drink high concentrated green tea for around 12 weeks can lose 0.44 pounds to 7.7 pounds more than those who don't drink the tea.

You should note that your green tea should have high amounts of antioxidants and catechins for you to lose weight. The two compounds increase your fat-burning capacity and metabolism.

One type of green tea that contains high amounts of antioxidants and catechins is Matcha. It is widely used for weight loss.

One matcha tea study found out that people who drink 3 grams of this type of tea per day burn a lot more fat during exercise than those who do not drink it.

Green tea also contains caffeine, a compound known to boost energy levels, improve exercise performance and promote weight loss.

4. Black Tea

Just like green tea, this type also contains substances that will promote weight loss.

During its manufacturing process, black tea undergoes more oxidation. It is exposed to air more than all the other types of tea. This results in a darker color and intense flavor.

Black tea contains high amounts of polyphenols. The drink also has a group of polyphonic substances known as flavonoids. Polyphenols have powerful antioxidant properties that will help you reduce your weight.

Scientists have shown that these black tea polyphenols can help you reduce your daily calorie intake, promote gut-friendly bacteria growth, and stimulate the breakdown of fats.

One study involving 111 subjects demonstrated how people who drank three cups of black tea every day for three months lost a lot more weight and reduced their waist circumference more than those in the control group.

5. Protein Drinks

Proteins are known to curb hunger, promote fullness and decrease appetite. These are essential factors if you are trying to lose weight.

Proteins do all these wonders by increasing hunger levels, reducing hormones such as GLP-1, and reducing ghrelin, a hormone responsible for appetite.

One study involving 90 overweight people found out that those who consumed 56g of proteins daily for 23 weeks lost about 2.3 kilograms of fat more than the control group who consumed no proteins.

Pea, hemp, and whey protein powders are some of the few varieties you can add to your drink, shakes, and smoothies to help you lose weight.

6. Apple Cider Vinegar

Taking apple cider vinegar is another way you can boost your weight loss rate every morning.

The substance contains acetic acid, which is known to stimulate weight loss. It does so by decreasing your insulin levels, suppressing your appetite, burning fats, and improving your metabolism.

Research in animals has shown that acetic acid can prevent weight gain and decrease fat accumulation in the liver and belly.

One study involving 144 obese subjects demonstrated how taking a beverage containing two tablespoons of vinegar every day could result in weight loss, reduced waist circumference, and belly.

According to NCBI, apple cider vinegar helps slow stomach emptying. This can reduce over-eating and make you feel fuller for an extended period.

Drinking acidic things such as apple cider vinegar can erode your teeth. This is why you should consume it in a controlled manner.

Here is how to drink apple cider vinegar for weight loss morning:

• Add two tablespoons (30ml) into a beverage of your choice.

• You can alternately take the two tablespoons directly. However, be sure to rinse your teeth with a lot of water to prevent them from eroding.

- Do not take more than two tablespoons in a day.

7. Water

Drinking a lot of water is one of the simplest yet helpful ways to improve your health and lose a lot of weight.

Taking a few water glasses will keep you feel between your meals, reduce the number of calories you take and increase the energy you burn daily.

Scientists say that taking water before any meal can go a long way in helping you cut on calorie consumption and shed off some pounds.

One research involving 48 overweight subjects found out that those who drank two glasses (500ml) of water before meals lost 44% more weight in 12 weeks than those who didn't drink water before eating.

Drinking cold water forces your body to burn a few calories to warm the liquid to body temperature. This will increase your rest energy expenditure and lead to weight loss.

One study involving 21 overweight kids found that resting energy could be increased by 25% for around 40 minutes after taking 10ml of cold water per kilogram of your body weight.

8. Coffee

Coffee is the best morning drink for weight loss.

People around the world widely use the beverage to lift moods and boost energy levels.

Coffee contains caffeine. The substance acts as a body stimulant and is responsible for weight loss.

When you take the drink in the morning, it will reduce your overall calorie intake for the day and boost your metabolism. This will result in weight loss.

One research involving 33 overweight subjects found out that those who took a coffee drink containing 6 milligrams of caffeine per kilogram consumed fewer calories than those who drank less or no caffeine.

If you take the beverage every morning, you will have an easier time maintaining your weight loss over time.

A study containing 2,500 subjects concluded that maintaining weight loss over time can be achieved by drinking more caffeinated drinks such as coffee.

9. Lemon Water

All you need in your glass every morning is freshly squeezed lemon juice to lose weight.

Here is how to drink lemon juice in the morning for weight loss:

• Squeeze fresh lemons into a glass

• Mix them with some hot water

• Add a half teaspoon of chia seeds.

• Add honey to taste.

After stirring the ingredients, what you will drink is a high protein drink. It will help you keep your stomach full and improve your body immunity.

Keeping away hunger rescues you from binging on those fast foods and fatty meals sold in the streets.

10. Detox Water

Detox water is an excellent drink that has the capabilities of purifying your body and increasing metabolism. This quickly leads to weight loss when you adopt a healthy lifestyle.

To prepare detox water:

- Add hot water into your glass.

- Add in sliced cucumbers in the glass.

- Squeeze a fresh lemon into the glass

- Add mint leaves and a slice of ginger.

- Leave it for about 10 minutes before consuming it.

Final Thought

Morning drinks for weight loss such as green tea and all the others listed above help boost metabolism, increase satiety, and minimize hunger. These factors are essential in weight loss.

Are Protein Shakes Good For Weight Loss

Weight gain and obesity are increasingly becoming a health risk to individuals in recent years, and the notion that those problems are caused by lack of willpower doesn't do any justice. Although weight gain is largely a product of eating behavior and lifestyle, some individuals are not entirely in control of their body size. Overweight and obesity can be caused by several factors, including genetics and hormones, making some people predisposed to gaining weight. Many turn to weight loss interventions such as workouts and protein shakes. So, are protein shakes good for weight loss?

Despite the predisposition to gain weight, people can overcome their genetic disadvantages by changing their lifestyle and behavior. It is not a simple task, but it can be accomplished through willpower, dedication, and perseverance. One of the most popular strategies for weight loss is to follow a high protein diet because protein curbs one's appetite, thus resulting in the reduction of the total calories consumed in a day.

What Are Protein Shakes?

Due to the importance they play or are perceived to play, the world of protein shakes is vast and does not seem to end. They come in different types, flavors, and formulations for any conceivable dietary need under the sun. Based on your preference, you can purchase premixed, ready-to-drink bottles, or protein powder.

The conception behind protein shakes is that they are meal replacements meant to help people lose weight. Because protein is filling, it may aid in suppressing your appetite by keeping in check your hunger hormones.

Most protein shakes for weight loss work by having a person replace either one or two meals per day with a shake, and then the third meal should be small and with low calories. In some extreme protein shakes diets, one drinks the shakes only for several days without any other food, but most professionals disapprove of this method.

The protein shakes can prove to be a valuable weight loss tool when consumed moderately. To be truly effective and healthy, they need to be paired with a couple of other sustainable lifestyle changes.

How Does The Protein Shake Diet Work?

To begin with, protein shakes offer more than just protein. Many manufacturers tend to fortify the shakes with a variety of vitamins and other minerals. Some may even have fruits, vegetables, and other essential nutrients. The important question here is, why are protein shakes good for weight loss?

A link has been established between the consumption of proteins and an increased feeling of fullness. It, therefore, follows that people who include enough protein in their daily diets ought to have fewer food cravings, and hence they will eat less. Some choose to get the protein through shakes. Below is a sample of a protein diet daily meal plan:

- Two protein shakes (between 200 and 300 calories each)

- Three small snacks (about 100 calories each)

- One full meal such as dinner (between 400 and 500 calories)

Based on this diet plan, the protein shakes are to be taken in the morning and at lunchtime. This is a very low calorie meal plan which should always be discussed with and monitored by a physician.

Are protein shakes for breakfast good for weight loss? There cannot be protein shakes as effective as the breakfast ones. This is because when you wake up, it is when you are hungry the most and will be tempted to eat a lot. Substituting your normal heavy breakfast with protein shakes already reduces the amount of food you eat. Most importantly, the protein shake will keep you feeling full. Hence you won't be craving more food.

When To Have Protein Shakes?

Another good time to consume a protein shake is after a workout. This is the point at which your body needs instant nourishment for muscle recovery and growth. The recommended consumption window is 30 to 45 minutes after your workout. This timeline is important because protein uptake is usually faster after a workout. You can also take the shake 30 minutes before your workout to energize yourself and boost your stamina.

How Good Are Protein Shakes for Weight Loss?

Are high protein shakes good for weight loss? When taken properly, protein shakes can be very effective in weight loss and control. That said, you must be aware that protein shakes alone are not the magic bullet for your body goals. Incorporate an overall healthy diet and a workout plan, and you will be amazed by the results. Below are some of the benefits of protein shakes to weight loss:

- Weight loss: Don't forget that the reason why you are drinking protein shakes in the first place is to lose weight. Getting enough protein is crucial in the weight loss journey and weight maintenance. Protein shakes achieve weight loss in several ways, including the fact that protein is more filling than carbs.

- Appetite control: Even people who are not keen on losing weight but have appetite problems can benefit from protein shakes. Protein is good for controlling appetite because it is dense and takes longer to digest. This means that you will remain full for much longer and wouldn't eat in that period. Protein also controls appetite by regulating ghrelin, which is the hunger hormone.

• Stable blood sugar levels: Protein can help stabilize your blood sugar levels. Sometimes blood sugar dips between meals, but it can be kept in check by the inclusion of a bit more protein in your meals.

• Building muscle: Intake of strategic supplementation with a protein, such as whey, can be good for muscle growth. Muscle growth is accelerated even more when you pair the protein with a resistance exercise. This will help your body to be leaner and have more stability (4).

- Metabolism: Protein works to increase the thermic effect of food. The thermic effect of food relates to the number of calories you burn by digesting what you eat. With an increased metabolism rate, your chances of losing weight are very high.

Risks And Side Effects

- Meal replacement shakes should not completely replace a healthy, balanced diet. Doing so could be harmful because there is no way you can get all the essential nutrients from just a single food source. You may end up losing more weight than you anticipated or even leave your body vulnerable to diseases.

- If the body does not get enough calories and nutrients, there is the risk that you might experience problems with metabolism. The result will be slowing or disrupting your weight loss plan. Furthermore, eating a varied diet reduces your chances of having obesity.

• A good number of protein shakes utilize large sweetener quantities to improve their flavor, and this can trigger blood sugar spikes.

• Consuming too much protein over the long term may not be good for your body. It may cause you problems in the kidneys and bones and even increase the risk of certain cancers.

• Some protein shakes contain unsafe levels of contaminants such as mercury, arsenic, lead, and cadmium. These contaminants can potentially cause serious health problems, some of which are life-threatening.

• Because they are nutritional supplements, protein shakes are not subject to stringent regulations, as is the case with medicine, and marketing materials of these products may sometimes be misleading.

Types Of Protein

There is no limit to the number of different protein options available in the market, so you have to figure one which is right for you. If you are lucky, you might find one that matches your Myers-Briggs personality type.

What protein shakes are good for weight loss? Here are some:

Whey

Whey is undoubtedly one of the most, if not the most, common and inexpensive type of protein. The protein is isolated from cow's milk and is readily absorbed. It is very efficient in building muscle, and the good thing about it is its availability. You can easily get it off any counter just in case you are experiencing a protein emergency.

Are whey protein shakes good for weight loss? Whey protein does not only help you gain muscle but also lose fat as well. However, it must be combined with exercise to see weight loss results.

Casein

This type of protein is also isolated from the milk of a cow, but it is not as effective in building muscle as whey. One other disadvantage is that it is a bit more expensive. Casein takes longer than whey to digest. This means it will keep you feeling full for a longer period, which is especially a good thing when you are trying to lose weight.

Egg

The egg-based protein powder is a good solid option for the liquid shake.

This type of protein has the upper hand because it is very easy for your body to absorb. The downside is that it is only made with the egg whites, hence, the consumers will be missing out on the many benefits of the yolk.

Soy

The good thing with protein shakes is that they accommodate even individuals who have gone vegan. Soy protein is among the best when it comes to plant-based diets because it is a complete protein. This means that soy protein contains all the essential amino acids that your body requires, just like with animal proteins.

There is a controversy surrounding soy because it has phytoestrogens, which allegedly have effects on hormones, although the overall body of scientific evidence suggests that soy is perfectly safe to consume.

Pea

Pea may be the subject of many juvenile jokes, but its protein is as good as any other plant-based protein. It is an alternative solid choice, especially for vegetarians. Although it is a complete protein, it is a little low in the amino acid methionine. Good thing that this can be quickly remedied by adding nut butter or nut milk to your pea protein shake, and you are good to go.

Hemp

As is the case with soy and pea, hemp is also a plant-based protein. It is also a complete protein. Another advantage of hemp is that it is a good source of healthy omega-3 fats. Its amino acid lysine content is slightly lower, a situation that can be rectified by adding tofu or almond butter to the hemp protein shake, or simply varying your plant protein sources from shake to shake or meal to meal.

Rice

Brown rice protein powder is one of the most common vegan protein choices. It is relatively cheap and happens to be a complete protein. It is similar to hemp due to its low lysine.

Homemade Protein Shakes For Weight Loss

Why buy protein shakes when you can make them at home? Sometimes you may not trust the protein shakes that are made in a factory, or you may not have the money to buy the shakes day after day. Worry not because there are several homemade protein shakes you can try.

But, are pure protein shakes good for weight loss? There are many benefits other than weight loss to be expected from the homemade protein shakes below:

Peanut butter protein shake

The homemade peanut butter protein shake gives you a nutty, creamy, and delicious feel. The upside with this shake is that it does not contain added sugar, and it is high in fiber and low in fat. Prepare it by blending 1 cup of yogurt, ½ cup of almond milk, 1 to 2 tablespoons of peanut butter, and 15-20 green grapes. Refrigerate the mixture and enjoy it chilled.

Chocolate and a banana protein shake

Chocolate! Are chocolate protein shakes good for weight loss? It may be unheard of, but chocolate and bananas do make a great combination and are also very good for weight loss. In addition to having great taste, they also make your protein shake super healthy. To prepare it, you need 10 almonds, ½ cup of yogurt, ¾ cup of milk, ½ teaspoon cinnamon, ¼ cup of cooked quinoa, 1 banana cut into chunks, and 1 tablespoon of cocoa powder. Blend the mixture in the blender.

Berry protein shake

All types of berries are efficient antioxidants and twice as a great source of fiber, which is important in your weight loss journey. You can opt to use strawberries, blackberries, or even gooseberries in your smoothie. The recipe includes 7-10 berries, ½ cup of whipped cottage cheese, ¼ cup of water, 1 tablespoon of chia seeds, and a little honey, but it is optional.

Vegan protein shake

Is plant-based protein shakes good for you for weight loss? Most plant-based protein shakes are complete proteins that make them a great alternative for individuals keen on losing some pounds. The vegan protein shake is designed for individuals who decided to stop the consumption of milk and dairy products but are still in need of a high protein shake for weight loss.

To make the vegan protein shake blend, you need ¾ cup of silken tofu, 1 cup of almond or cashew milk, 1 banana, ¼ cup of cooked oats, 1 teaspoon of honey (or agave or other syrup), and 1 teaspoon of vanilla essence for flavor.

Raw egg protein shake

The raw egg protein shake is not only important for weight loss but also muscle building. The main ingredient of the homemade protein shake is raw egg, and you must ensure that the eggs you use are of good quality. The shake is made by mixing 1 raw egg including its yolk, ½ avocado, ½ cup of milk or coconut milk, 1 banana, 1 teaspoon of honey, and ½ teaspoon of cinnamon. To prepare, place all the ingredients in a blender and blend them.

Spinach flax protein shake

It is a green homemade shake prepared by combining 1 cup of unsweetened almond milk or any other kind of milk, spinach leaves, ½ cup of mango chunks, ½ cup of pineapple bits, ½ banana, 1 tablespoon of flax seeds, and 1 tablespoon of chia seeds. Blend the mixture and serve immediately.

Important Considerations

• Before you commence on a protein shake diet, reflect on whether you can manage your daily schedule if you eat just one meal per day. Remember that a protein shake isn't a meal but merely a meal replacement. Your body system may go into shock from eating three meals per day to drinking two of them. Another option would be to consume a normal 3-meal per day diet and include protein shakes as pre- or post-workout snacks.

- Also, take into consideration the duration you can or should use shakes as meal replacements. A moderate diet will enable you to lose about 1 to 2 pounds per week. This will determine the period in which you keep the diet going based on the number of pounds you intend to lose. Losing weight more quickly than this is not healthy or sustainable, so make sure you are consuming enough calories every day to nourish and fuel your body.

- The diet can only be successful if the snacks you incorporate and the daily meal(s) are nutritious and healthy.

You do not want your body to become weak due to poor dietary choices. It goes without saying that if the snacks or meals are not nutritious, then the results will not be as desired.

• Even though you will be on protein shakes, you will have to continue shopping for some groceries. That aside, you must establish that you have the willpower to stick to the diet plan. After taking the shake, you will probably feel that you haven't eaten what you are used to eating.

- You will need a lot of courage to avoid other unhealthy snack foods, especially if your workplace or home environment is filled with those foods. It won't make any sense to drink protein shakes once or twice a day and then overeat the rest of the time.

The Bottom Line

Are protein shakes good for weight loss? Many people have been in a place where they wondered if the before-and-after photos on some of the protein shake ads are legit. One of the reasons why protein shakes are very popular is because they are super convenient, and all one has to do is drink them. The good thing is that there is a lot of information available on how to use them efficiently. However, even though protein shakes have some benefits that may result in weight loss, they alone cannot guarantee weight loss.

Diets are great, but your body will thank you if you supplement your healthy nutrition plan with a good workout. Take up this 20 Min Full Body Workout at Home.